"Mental illness is not a choice or an excuse, but ignorance is."

"There is no shame in being open and honest about illnesses that affect millions of everyday people. Everyone has a certain degree of mental illness, but those who are dismissive would rather judge or question those who have chosen to openly share about their illness."-Kait

Gain hope, support, and victory!

A book created to provide hope, support, and insight to those who are affected by bipolar disorder and mental illness; Also including support and educational information for caregivers and loved ones. This site was not set up by a licensed professional in any way. I am just a fellow bipolar survivor and stigma fighter who believes that we all have the potential to gain control over our illnesses and win the battle.

"There is still hope for a more joyous and stronger future. Keep weathering the storm, push through the strength of the tides, take your time, relax, and breathe. Don't let the strong winds knock you down. Get up, fight, and try again. You are strong enough. Keep pressing on, embrace the moment, and never give up. Life is a beautiful journey. In time, you will see. " -Kait S.

Living with bipolar disorder or any mental illness can make it seem as though life is impossible, unfair, or feel as though one's life has been completely taken away from them at times. One also may feel like they can never win over their illness or even begin to know what feels real to them anymore. These are normal feelings to experience when having a mental illness such as bipolar disorder.

Bipolar disorder is considered a mental illness where those affected with the disorder will experience alternating periods of elation (mania) and depression. Not one person will experience bipolar disorder in the same way as another person will. Everyone who lives with bipolar disorder has their own set of symptoms, triggers, and will even react very differently to medications than others might. This makes sense because everybody in this world is different. We are all "wired" and put together in our own, unique ways. We all deal with symptoms of depression, stress, anxiety, and mania differently. With having a diagnosis that is similar to others such as "bipolar" or "depression," we will most certainly still have very similar feelings, worries, and struggles to others, but nothing is ever exact.

I have personally lived with bipolar my whole life and was first diagnosed at the young age of twelve. Over time, I began to accept the diagnosis of bipolar. It wasn't until early 2011 that I had decided to help others who also struggle with mental illnesses by providing them with knowledge, support, and hope that I had discovered in myself over the years.

Acceptance is the very first step to recover from any problem. I spent many years in therapy and with my psychiatrist gaining more knowledge of the disorder and treatment options. I learned about many coping methods and how to continue to talk openly about my feelings and illness. I found that when I had talked with my therapists over the years, I started to better understand myself and what I was going through. It has given me great comfort just knowing and having that reassurance that the feelings that I am or had been feeling are normal. It is very important for those with bipolar disorder or mental illness to keep communication open at all times. Communication is a much-needed and very helpful skill for those with bipolar to have if they want to successfully gain control over their illness. It is very important that the person struggling with the illness is able to open up to someone who they can trust when they have noticed sudden changes in their moods. I would also recommend to caregivers to approach and check in on their bipolar loved ones every so often and ask questions such as (but not limited to) "How are you feeling today?" "Can I help you with something?" or "Let's talk about it." Sometimes just being there and providing support for someone who is struggling can instantly change how they feel. The caregivers and the loved ones of a bipolar patient can make a great difference too. With every little bit of help, the journey to stability can become even more possible!

Always remember: You are never alone. We are all in this together to fight, survive, and conquer mental illness. We have the power to be our best selves and to begin to view the world differently and more positively than ever before. We are also here to fight the stigma that is attached to mental illness and show those who hold the judgments so closely that we are people too and that we have just as much potential as anyone else. We all deserve a chance at equality and happiness. We are stronger than the stigma!

Keep weathering the storm. Keep pushing forward and hold on for that chance for a much better tomorrow. You deserve it and you can do it!

"I have a mental illness. Does this make me a bad person?"

The answer is no. Mental illness does not define who a person is and it is not fair to think you (or anyone struggling) is a "bad" person for it. Like I have said before, the stigma attached to mental illness is unfair and I believe everyone should become more aware and be more open-minded about it. No one can choose what they are born with or how their brain functions. I have seen sadly, that there is more ignorance than understanding on these topics.

A lot of people who become diagnosed with a mental illness think they are an inadequate person or the parents may think "What did I do wrong?" or "What am I doing wrong?" No one is doing anything wrong and no one is in the wrong. No one would choose to struggle.

Something to think about: If someone mentions they have diabetes, heart disease, or epilepsy etc, are you understanding about their illness (and support them) or do you step aside? Mental illness is considered along the same lines as a physical illness and must be treated as one as well. It isn't just an emotional or behavioral trait or illness. It's a brain disorder. It isn't really all that different from a physical illness because it can affect physical functioning as well, but the stigma is there and made to see mental illness as a negative and it is and has been constantly misunderstood.

An example; In the times when my moods and emotions are out of control, I honestly just want support and understanding to get me through. I personally never try to do anything or act a certain way on purpose. Sometimes there is some "attention seeking," but this does not make me a bad person. In times like these, I feel scared and frustrated inside and I worry I'll lose control. Sometimes I do actually lose control and fall apart because it becomes too much to keep festered up inside. Most times I don't want to go through those days or moments alone and I shouldn't have to.

It's honestly a scary feeling and I can bet people who struggle with other physical illnesses etc. feel scared when their illness is suddenly out of control too.

Please be open-minded and show some love, ignorance hurts. Everyone deserves to feel and be accepted/loved.

Why Judge Those Who Live With Mental Illness?

Why judge those who are "different"? Are they less human than anyone else? Do they not deserve the same respect? Do some people just judge out of the fear of their own insecurities? Is it just easier to dismiss everything and pretend?

I think and analyze a lot about how and why certain things happen. These types of questions and behaviors constantly have me (and probably many others) stumped as to why others choose to judge those who are different from them.

Why has mental illness become something that we can't or that we are not supposed to talk about? Some see mental illness better kept as a "secret." They might believe that it would be better for those types of issues to be left unsaid and to never be brought up or dealt with. They might also believe by not talking about mental illness or by recognizing the issue, that they are probably doing the person struggling with the illness a favor. In reality, those who have chosen to dismiss mental illness and avoid the topic completely may only be avoiding and helping one person. **Themselves.** Not necessarily the person struggling with the mental illness. Those with such reactions may feel awkward, ashamed, or embarrassed that these types of issues are so close to them.

They might say things like or similar to, "No, don't mention that! Shh! We don't want to talk about so and so and their struggles with mental illness."

When people have this type of reaction or treat mental illness as a horrible or god-awful thing, it comes off as if they are ashamed or embarrassed of the mentally ill. These reactions and attitudes towards mental illness ultimately hurts those who struggle every day with mental illness. Especially if these types of reactions are ones that happen within the family or from those who are close to us. Did you know that there are different characteristics and types of mental illness in every family and everyone? From stress, to anxiety, to depression, and schizophrenia? **Every** person has and is going to experience some type of mental illness in their lifetime. Mental illness is **not** as rare as we once thought and it should **never** be considered as a sign of weakness.

A quote I wrote (modified): "Mental illness is **not** a choice or an excuse, but ignorance is."

Those who suffer from mental illness are not choosing to suffer and it is not possible for them to just change their thinking or "snap out of it." It takes a great deal of understanding and support towards those who live with a mental illness for them to feel accepted as they should always and already be. As mental illness becomes more common and as the public begins to accurately recognize what mental illness is and does, they may no longer see mental illness as a weakness or a flaw. The fear and misunderstanding may be lifted from those who aren't familiar with such illnesses and also from those who are struggling. Everyone should keep an open mind, listen without judging, and educate themselves further about mental illness. If we successfully recognize, understand, and accept the struggles of those who live with a mental illness, we might successfully conquer and overcome the unnecessary stigma that is attached to mental illness.

Bipolar Disorder and Relationships. Can a Person With Bipolar Have a Successful Relationship?

It has been contemplated whether or not relationships can be successful if an individual has bipolar disorder. I personally believe that individuals who have bipolar disorder, or any mental illness for that matter, have the same amount of risk in relationships as those who do not live with a mental illness. Here's why:

First of all, most people who live with mental illness, myself included, tend to have a negative self-image which can make them ultimately feel undesirable and develop constant worries and fears in relationships, …but guess what? People who don't live with a mental illness can have those very same feelings and worries in relationships and in general too. As I've mentioned many times before, we are never alone in the ways we feel. It's human to have feelings and emotions, but look at it this way, people with bipolar disorder tend to feel those emotions at a different extremity and more often. This doesn't mean that people with bipolar can't be involved in successful or happy relationships even though there may be very difficult and strenuous times, but this is true with any couple. Same goes for the bipolar disorder and having children debate as well. As humans, even with a mental illness, we have the potential and the right to be involved in relationships and have children. The debate whether or not individuals with mental illness are capable to successfully be in relationships or have children should not be an issue. They are still capable of being good spouses and parents. Those who don't have a mental illness have the same amount of risk of making mistakes in relationships and in parenting. We are all human.

With bipolar disorder, individuals tend to experience periods of alternating highs and lows often referred to as mania and depression (manic-depression). Some people may be wondering or are curious as to why people with bipolar disorder may struggle in relationships. Well, there may be a few factors that relate with the mania and depression that cause symptoms which can make being in relationships a bit more difficult.

Some factors (but not limited to) that may affect relationships may be:

- = advice for the partners of a bipolar

spouse/boyfriend/girlfriend

-Excessive spending – Mania can cause times where those with the disorder may want to spend more money and this may even greatly affect a bank account negatively, worsen mood problems (guilt, depression, regret, sadness), and ultimately it can affect the relationship. Mania can also cause hyper sexuality, rapid and excessive speech, and irritability.

- -When the partner of a bipolar individual notices any signs of mania and/or excessive spending, he or she should take control of the money (credit cards, check books, cash, etc) and also notify their doctor and/or document the mood changes noticed just to be safe. This also applies to other types of mood changes. It helps people with bipolar to have a responsible and understanding partner who can help support them when they experience the mood changes.

-Mood swings/Anxiety – With the constant mood changes it can be very difficult to have a smooth sailing relationship without conflict. All relationships, no matter who you are, are going to experience conflict. With bipolar disorder, they often have times where they feel irritable, angry, emotional, and also have times of mania (euphoria- elevated hyper mood) and sometimes for no apparent reason or cause. Sometimes the trigger can be identified, but sometimes there are moods where everything flips the switch the wrong way seemingly without cause. There are also many moments where a person with bipolar may lash out in anger such as throwing objects, hitting, crying/screaming, and saying/yelling hurtful things. This can make for a very frustrating and rocky relationship without the right strategies to control it.

- It is important that the partner can help redirect him/her when the bipolar individual is experiencing mood swings and or obsessive thoughts. It may be helpful to have a partner that knows when to help the person struggling with mood swings or worries calm down appropriately, but also knows the times when to walk away from behaviors (attention-seeking etc). Sometimes staying around while he or she is experiencing a mood swing can also make matters worse. The key is to know **when**, because there are times where things could go horribly wrong. When its noticeable that the bipolar partner is starting to get irritable, is yelling/screaming, throwing things, etc, it is best to try to catch these mood changes very early to prevent it from escalating any further, if possible. There are times where they may say or yell hurtful things that may possibly make you second guess or become really frustrated or angry in your relationship. It is important to keep in mind, for the sake of the relationship and sanity, that these moments do not last forever and more than likely the bipolar individual is just having a mood swing and isn't meaning to anger you or upset you. *Sometimes* a good strategy would be to ask them "Talk to me about it.", "What's bothering you?", "How can I help?", "What would make you feel better?" ,"Let's go find something enjoyable to do.", etc. More than likely your bipolar spouse would love your attention, know that you are listening, and they can see you care. **Support is huge** for those struggling to have in their lives.

Advice to those in a relationship with a person who has bipolar disorder: Research! Research! Research! Learn about the disorder, go to doctors' appointments, and listen to them. Also, observe and get to know them both inside and out. Know what their triggers are and recognize the mood changes. This is very important advice.

Lastly, the key to making a relationship work when someone struggles with a mental illness would be ultimately to have the right person by their side who they know will **support and understand** them- that is key. Someone who is open-minded, patient, dependable, willing to listen, and who is willing to help them. Also, **communication** is essential. I cannot express that enough- that is also a key to *any* successful relationship. A lot of common mistakes in relationships is not being with the right person. This is true for everyone including those without mental illness. If it's not the right person, the relationship, but most importantly the mental and emotional health of each individual, will be negatively impacted causing more complications.

In closing, can a person with bipolar disorder have successful relationships? YES, yes they can! It is a matter of having the right person, both being aware of any sudden mood changes, and patience. Patience is also a huge helpful factor in relationships.

Never give up thinking that a person who has bipolar disorder means they cannot have successful relationships. It is possible, but it takes time and patience as it does for *everyone*.

Keep your head up and always be good to yourself.

The Struggle: Bipolar Disorder and Working

When a person struggles with bipolar disorder, it can often be very difficult for them to follow through with daily tasks and routines that most are capable and used to doing on a daily basis. Holding a job and working is one of them. This can be a huge road block for those who struggle with the disorder mentally, emotionally, and financially.

The fact that many with bipolar disorder cannot work is often judged and constantly misunderstood. They may hear comments such as, but not limited to:

- "Why can't so and so work?"
- "What is so difficult about going to work?"
- "What does bipolar disorder have to do with it?"
- "It's laziness. There is no reason you aren't able

to work or hold a job."

- "Everyone is expected to work. There is no reason you can't."

It is also a fact that those who make such comments are unfamiliar and uneducated about the illness.

In fact, there are many factors that make carrying out daily tasks difficult and strenuous on a bipolar individual. There are many symptoms of the disorder that contribute and that can cause disruption in their daily lives.

If unfamiliar with bipolar disorder, bipolar is a chemical imbalance in the brain characterized as alternating mood changes (*also known as mood swings*) of mania and depression. Bipolar is often referred to now as a physical illness and *not just* a mental illness because it can also affect their lives physically as well. For example, their energy levels which can greatly affect their ability to accomplish and carry out those daily tasks.

During mania, a person living with the disorder may exhibit an increase in energy, excessive or rapid speech, insomnia, spending sprees, irritability, aggression, and an overall seemingly hyper and/or agitated personality.

During depression, an individual living with the disorder may present common depression symptoms such as, a decrease in energy, sadness, withdrawn behavior, aggression, irritability, feelings of hopelessness and/or abandonment (lonely), crying, anxiety, suicidal thoughts or ideations, and negative self-image, thoughts, and thinking patterns.

Even with the mood changes between mania and depression, bipolar individuals also can and do experience some "normal" states which often require treatment of mood stabilizers, antidepressants, and/or anti-psychotic medications from a licensed psychiatrist.

Now this still may raise questions about how these mood changes can affect a person living with bipolar disorder so greatly. With these drastic mood changes, a person who lives with bipolar disorder emotions, mentality, and overall appearance both physically and mentally changes.

In times of mania, the individual may be unusually productive which actually can be very helpful when working a job and completing daily tasks. They may describe these feelings as *"I have never been feeling better."* and *"life is great!"* After the mania starts to develop and swing into a depression state, the individual may start to feel and appear too overstimulated which can lead into the anxiety, irritability, and aggression. Once the over-stimulation stage occurs, it may suddenly become very difficult for them to concentrate and finish up the task they were currently attending to without becoming frustrated, irritable, and overwhelmed.

In times of depression, individuals with bipolar disorder may feel unmotivated, a decrease in energy levels, an overall sadness, and unhappiness in their lives. Some may describe these feelings and episodes as, *"I'm bored with my life." "Noting matters anymore." No one cares about me." Things would just be easier if I wasn't around."* There are times where the depression becomes too low to even function at all. With depression, it is common for them to feel apathetic towards life. The feelings of hopelessness, sadness, the negative thoughts/worries, and unusually low energy levels can sometimes result in more serious complications such as suicide.

In a work environment, it can be **very difficult** to cope with the severity of the symptoms. At work, most people tend to try to be on their best behaviors. Bipolar individuals strive to do the same. When they are at work and are experiencing such severe and sudden changes in their moods and symptoms, it may become way too overwhelming to cope with both the stress of the work, the overall environment (feelings of discomfort and lack of support), and the changes they are currently experiencing within themselves. With all of this happening at once, this can very easily create a recipe for disaster causing the individual to leave or skip work , quit, and/or even result in a termination in employment. When bipolar individuals start repeating the patterns of quitting or being terminated from a job, it may be a good idea to create or turn to a safety net such as <u>SSI</u>, <u>SSDI</u>, or other sources of income/support.

- <u>Social Security Disability Resource Site</u>
- <u>Is Bipolar Disorder a disability according to</u>

Social Security?
- Social Security Disability: SSI For Bipolar Disorder

It is very important for those who struggle with bipolar disorder to be properly medicated, have regular doctors appointments, and to ultimately be stable before setting out to work. It is also **true** that there are many successful working bipolar individuals who can go to work daily. This article may definitely be a *not-all* statement. Some factors that possibly make it more possible for them to **succeed in their work environment** would be:

- The type of job. Something not too stressful and/or something they enjoy doing.
- The job setting or the environment.
- Having an understanding employer.
- The amount of hours or the shifts.
- Successful, while on-the-job coping techniques.
- Seeing a therapist and psychiatrist often.
- Stabilized moods – Having the correct and working medications.

So, what's the deal?

People with mental illness and bipolar disorder require a little more understanding and support. It's not that they don't want to work or because they are lazy, it's because of a chemical imbalance in the brain that greatly and ultimately affects their daily lives. It can become very frustrating and stressful for the bipolar individual not being able to

work when they really want it. It can affect their self-esteem and their personal life as well. Working is definitely an obstacle for some bipolar individuals, but we've learned there is always hope and there are always more tries and options. Never give up and always believe in yourself.

Encouraging Thoughts, Reminders, And Inspirations

If you have been having a rough time lately or are just in need of that little boost of inspiration and hope, I would like to share some with you today. Also, this post can be helpful to those who wish to increase their knowledge and understanding further. Here are some random, but important points I have made and wrote regarding mental illnesses. I thought I'd share them hoping they can be of some help to others and provide some insight as well.

Here are some helpful tools and points I would like to share:

- Each time we fall to the ground, we always gain experience and learn more about ourselves. Strategies to make us stronger. We understand what it feels like to be on top of the world and at the very worst. I'm pretty sure we have felt just about every emotion possible and that can be a truly great gift. Not everyone gets to view or experience these types of feelings.

- Mental illness has become something that we just don't talk about. A "secret." Heck, we NEED to talk about it. Keep an open mind, listen, and accept.
- Bipolar does NOT mean you have two different personalities and it is NOT a personality flaw by any means.
- Bipolar Disorder can't really be something you "recover" from, but more of a survival/fight or improvement. Wouldn't you agree?
- First step to stability and treatment is to admit to or recognize the problem & find a solution. Take control- You are stronger than the problem.
- Living with a mental illness offers greater insight and compassion.
- I've noticed in times where I'm not doing so well, I've said repeatedly, "I don't want to feel like this anymore." That is the time I choose to **do** something about it.

- Sometimes you just have to wake up and tell yourself "I'm going to have a good day. I deserve it."
- Laughing is one of my favorite things to do. Make it a priority in your own life and watch your happiness grow.
- Laugh and smile even when you don't feel like it because that is when you really need it. Try it out!
- Life is full of ups and downs, but it's worth every second of them. You only live once. Keep

moving forward, feel the moment, and enjoy.

- "You are never given more than you can handle" and I strongly believe that.
- Everyday is a new day. Enjoy today for what it is and try not to dwell on tomorrow.
- I notice I tend to tell myself to calm down a lot and other things like "It will be okay, Kait." I do this a lot and it sometimes helps with anxiety. Try it out for yourself. Always treat yourself well.
- Avoiding or ignoring something doesn't make it just go away.
- Do the things you've always wanted to do. Be yourself. Don't live to please others, but show respect. No one is as perfect as they may seem. Therefore, no one should expect anyone else to be.
- The only person who can fix and make you feel better is YOU.
- If you begin having feelings of hopelessness, remind yourself that you are strong enough to work through it and that things always get better.
- Just think- Things could always be worse. Somewhere in the world, others have it much worse than you right now. Breathe in, breathe out. Be grateful for all the things accomplished and the strengths – try not to focus on "faults."
- Referring to relationships: One of the worst things you can do is try to make yourself believe that you are happy when inside it's killing you.

Been there, done that. Never settle for less than YOU deserve. Trust me, it will be worth it.

- Everyone deserves equality… EVERYONE.
- I can be over emotional, an over-thinker, filled with overwhelming amounts of anxiety, but I'm a person just like you. Fight the stigma!
- NOT ALL people who live with bipolar or other mental illnesses lie, cheat, steal, spend tons of money, do drugs, drink, are addicts, hurt themselves ,or are violent. Break the stigma!

Inspiring quotes from some inspiring people to make your day a bit brighter:

"I don't think of all the misery, but of all the beauty that still remains." – Anne Frank

"I believe that every person is born with talent." -Maya Angelou

"Being ignorant is not so much a shame, as being unwilling to learn." ~Benjamin Franklin

"Listen to your intuition. You will be amazed at what you already know."

"We need to consider how our actions, in affecting the environment, are likely to affect others."

"It is a very hard undertaking to seek to please everybody." – Publilius Syrus

"Let my heart beat louder, let my heart speak louder than my head" -Louder lyrics by Charice

"Whatever you are, be a good one."

"If someone woke up in the middle of an operation, it would hurt a fair bit. Unfortunately, therapy doesn't have anesthetic – use self-care."

"If we're growing, we're always going to be out of our comfort zone." ~ John Maxwell

"It is of immense importance to learn to laugh at ourselves." – Katherine Mansfield

"He who controls others may be powerful, but he who has mastered himself is mightier still." -Lao-Tzu

"Criticism, like rain, should be gentle enough to nourish a man's growth without destroying his roots." -Frank Clark

"If you want to conquer fear, don't sit at home and think about it. Go out and get busy." – Andrew Carnegie

"Take your life in your own hands and what happens? A terrible thing: no one to blame." – Erica Jong

"When you get to the end of your rope, tie a knot & hang on." -Franklin D. Roosevelt

"Give love and unconditional acceptance to those you encounter, and notice what happens." – Wayne Dyer

"Minds are like parachutes – they only function when open." -Thomas Dewar

"The reason people give up so fast is because they tend to look at how far they still have to go instead of how far they have gotten."

"Nothing in life is to be feared. It is only to be understood." – Marie Curie

"Life throws the bad things at us to make the good things all the more worthwhile."

"Absurdity and anti—absurdity are the two poles of creative energy." — Karl Lagerfeld

"Clear your energy, honor your rhythm, live your vision " — George Denslow

"It's not your job to like me – it's mine." – Byron Katie

"I think the next best thing to solving a problem is finding some humor in it"~ Frank Howard Clark

"Cling to your imperfections… They're what makes you unique."

"Intellectuals solve problems; geniuses prevent them." -Albert Einstein

"Forgive yourself for your faults and your mistakes and move on." – Les Brown

"Above all things, never be afraid. The enemy who forces you to retreat is himself afraid of you at that very moment." ~ Andre Maurois

"We must hurt in order to grow, fail in order to know, and lose in order to gain. Because some lessons in life, are best learned through pain."

"If you believe deep down you're bad, have baggage, unlovable, others will say-she knows herself better than anyone,who am I to argue?"-Dr. Phil

"Never be bullied into silence. Never allow yourself to be made a victim. Accept no one's definition of your life" -Harvey Fierstein

"Instead of being positive or negative, right or wrong, I strive to simply be AUTHENTIC." -Mastin Kipp

"Don't let your ears "witness" what your eyes didn't see and don't let your mouth speak what your heart doesn't feel."

"It's easy to tell someone to face their fears, but until you put yourself in their shoes, you wouldn't understand."

Bipolar Disorder And Having Children

If you are still rather young and you have a mental illness such as bipolar disorder, the ability to have children may have crossed your mind.

This can be a very debatable topic, but I personally see it as a personal choice and it also depends highly on the individual's health. If you or your spouse has bipolar disorder and would like to have children, it is definitely something you both should look into and talk about with your doctors to see if it is possible for you. I don't see any reason why someone with the disorder should not be allowed or should not be able to have a child unless some medical factors lay in that may affect your health negatively. With having a diagnosis such as bipolar disorder, there may be some concerns you have about having children. I will be upfront and honest, there are several factors I see to consider before just going about it.

1. **Have a plan**. When you have bipolar disorder, it is a very important and beneficial to your health to plan ahead with your spouse and doctors before becoming pregnant.

2. **Bipolar disorder is genetic.** The disorder can be passed down from parent to child, but that does NOT mean your child will necessarily develop the disorder. It's a chance. *According to the site* ScienceDaily *"children of parents with bipolar disorder had an increased risk of having a bipolar spectrum disorder (41 or 10.6 percent vs. two or 0.8 percent) and having any mood or anxiety disorder. Children in families where both parents had bipolar disorders also were more likely than those in families containing one parent with bipolar disorder to develop the condition (four of 14 or 28.6 percent vs. 37 of 374 or 9.9 percent); however, their risk for other psychiatric disorders was the same as offspring of one parent with bipolar disorder."*

3. **Most medications should NOT be used during pregnancy.** If you are currently medicated, you may, most likely, have to stop your medications during the pregnancy or look into an alternate treatment. Also, if you plan on breast-feeding, most medications are not safe to use

during that time. You may have to seek out other options or plan ahead with your doctor.

4. **Expect or prepare for possible extreme body and mood changes during and after giving birth.**Pregnancy changes a woman's body drastically during pregnancy due to hormone changes, increase in blood, emotions, and the overall mental and physical well-being bipolar or not. This can disrupt and often make the bipolar illness worsen due to all the chemical, hormonal, and bodily changes during and after pregnancy. It is very important to take extra care of yourself and keep in touch with your doctors and a therapist.You may have heard about postpartum depression before and that is good – It's good to be aware of this condition and be conscious of any changes you may notice within your body. Postpartum depression or postpartum psychosis is *possible*, but not a definite outcome. This may be a risk to talk to your partner and doctor about before deciding if having children is for you. *According to* PubMed Health, *"Postpartum depression is moderate to severe depression in a woman after she has given birth. It may occur soon after delivery or up to a year later. Most of the time, it occurs within the first 3 months after delivery." From* Pregnancyinfo.net, *women who have a family history of psychosis, bipolar disorder or schizophrenia have a greater chance of developing the disorder. Additionally, women*

who have had a past incidence of postpartum psychosis are between 20% and 50% more likely of experiencing it again in a future pregnancy."

5. **Children, especially young infants, require a lot of attention and your time.** Children need a lot of attention and a positive role model. There are some, but definitely not all, that may not realize just how much attention they require and how important it is to be a great role model to their children. I am not saying that those who have bipolar disorder can't be good parents, give them the attention they need, or be a great role model. Those with bipolar disorder, like I have said before, can be just as good of parents as any other person out there. It just takes the right situation, precautions, support (spouse, family, doctors, etc), and extra time planning ahead.

   When you have an illness such as bipolar disorder, it is common for the illness to interfere with one's daily lives consisting of alternating moods, symptoms/behaviors, and emotions. The illness can consume a lot of one's time and take out a lot of energy in one's life. Some days it may feel as if there is no escape from the symptoms. A lot of personal space and down time is often necessary for those who live with bipolar and it's often difficult to put others needs before one's own. When it comes to children, they need and depend on you everyday. It may be quite strenuous when trying to take care of another person when you're in need of some personal space to cope and regroup. Something to consider would be to figure out a plan how it will be possible to take care of a child, but also cope with the disorder.

Essential tips if you are planning to have children:

- First, make sure your health is stable and under control. Talk with your spouse and doctor about medications, what to expect, and how to take care of yourself and the child.
- Second, have a working, successful plan. Make sure you plan out before you become pregnant and also for during and after the pregnancy. Always keep communication open – talk to your spouse and doctors frequently. Note any changes, even minor ones and report them back to your doctor and spouse. Also, have more than one plan if possible. This will increase your chances for a safer pregnancy and health if one plan ends up not working or something happens to change.
- As with any person before a pregnancy, consider your health, relationship, decide and plan on appropriate ways to cope around your child, and your overall feelings towards becoming a parent. Make sure you and your spouse are both ready and can support each other. Prepare for the worst, but don't expect it or worry about it. Just be prepared and keep an open mind.
- Create ways you can minimize stress and relax. Remaining stress-free as possible and being

relaxed is also very important. For example; Get plenty of rest, take breaks as needed, listen to soothing music, take a warm bath, light some candles, and keep coping skills (such as breathing exercises) close at hand. These are some ways to relax and keep your health and the stress under control.

Bipolar Disorder requires a lot of support, knowledge, and understanding. It is a plus if you and your spouse are aware of your symptoms, triggers, and frequency of episodes. Knowing and being aware of this can be a great help before planning a pregnancy.

From a personal point of view on the topic:
I am currently in my mid-twenties and I realize I am still young and have some time ahead to really think about having a family. Having children and wondering about my ability to be a good mother and wife has crossed my mind very frequently. I have definitely wanted to be a mom since a very young age, but I have also been unsure when in times of depression and despair. I know at times my bipolar disorder completely takes control over my life and I can feel as though everything is out of my hands. I have times where I am incredibly selfish where I need (or want) extreme amounts of attention. I am very protective and tend to get jealous easily. I wouldn't want these issues I struggle with to come between a child and I or make my

relationship with a spouse even more complicated. I fear for that. I fear that the relationship between a spouse and I would change drastically and we wouldn't have the closeness that we do now. I fear that I will lose all sense of comfort and control. I worry that I wouldn't be able to care for my child and give them the life they deserve. I worry and don't want my disorder to neglect the child or a spouse. I am also concerned and aware about the risks of my child developing a mood or anxiety disorder. It does worry me, but even with all the concerns revolving around my illness and my relationship, I know that deep down I really want to have a family. I know that being aware of my illness and worries will definitely help me when the time comes. I really think having a child is personal choice even if you struggle with a mental illness. I think anyone with a mental illness has just as much potential to be a great parent as anyone else. Every parent, no matter who you are, will make mistakes and that is also something to keep in mind too.

I also know that it is very important to be healthy first and ready for anything that may need to be faced later (and that may even mean waiting a bit longer if the time isn't right at that moment.) One benefit that keeps me going is if bipolar is passed down to my child, I would have the understanding of what they are going through. I would be able to relate to and understand my child. I know there are some parents that would love to understand their children and what they are going through better. I think this can be a fantastic benefit, but ultimately I would want my child to be healthy as possible and not have to go through the struggles I have. As of now, I am not even close to be planning for a family, but the thoughts do occasionally cross my mind about being bipolar and having children and I thought I should share.

Recognizing the Signs and Symptoms of Bipolar Disorder In Children and Adolescents

It has been said that spotting and diagnosing bipolar disorder in children and adolescents is often quite difficult for parents and physicians to accomplish. In general, bipolar disorder is a complicated illness that is not easily diagnosed and is often misdiagnosed in many cases.

As a person who was diagnosed with bipolar disorder as a child, I can understand and recognize the signs and symptoms of early on-set bipolar disorder. Please keep in mind that I am not a licensed professional in any way and this information should not be used for diagnostic purposes. Please contact your local physician or a pediatric psychiatrist for an evaluation if you have any suspicions. I decided to post this information to help anyone who would like to know a bit more about the bipolar symptoms I had recognized in children and adolescents.

Signs and Symptoms of Child and Adolescent Bipolar Disorder

- Insomnia- Not able to sleep at night. The child may feel more "awake" or "wired" at late hours of the night. As a child with bipolar, I used to stay up all night playing with my toys. I had a difficult time going to sleep and sticking to routine.
- Nightmares or Terrors- Some children may experience terrifying or vivid nightmares. Sometimes the dreams are said to be rather gory or out of the norm.
- Anxiety- This was a big symptom as a child. I was always anxious, felt restless, wasn't easily soothed, and I was a constant worrier.
- Separation Anxiety- Though I don't know if this would be considered a common characteristic of bipolar, but I had terrible separation anxiety and could be very clingy to the adults/caregivers in my life.
- Racing Thoughts- The thoughts just never stop. Thoughts full of creative ideas, images, worries, and all the above.

- Excitability- The child may appear unusually (extremely) silly to the point where it may be difficult to calm them down. An unusual silliness.
- Over-stimulation- After being around a large group of people or after a day with many things happening at once, the child may become overstimulated and exhibit tantrums or crying spells that seem unusual.
- Overactive Imagination and Creativity- (I see this as a gift of mental illness in general). The child may have an outstanding imagination and is extremely creative and/or gifted.
- Constipation or Tummy Troubles- This may seem like an odd symptom of bipolar disorder, but I am discovering that many children will experience stomach issues with a diagnosis such as bipolar disorder. In addition, many anxious children, due to the anxiety, struggle to have regular bowel movements.
- Colicky as a baby or an infant- Very difficult or impossible to soothe.
- Difficulty Concentrating or Staying Focused- Jumping from one thing or topic to another rapidly.
- Rapid Speech
- Unusual Sadness
- Feelings of Worthlessness or Guilt
- Low-Self-Esteem
- Sudden Mood Changes or Shifts- Happy and

joyful one minute, feelings of sadness and tearfulness the next with no apparent reason or cause.
- Thoughts or Talks of Death or Suicide
- Intrusive Thoughts- Unusual and scary thoughts that scare the child such as doing something that would harm others or themselves.
- Rage- The child may have little or no control over his or her emotions. The child may become easily angered over little things.

Reasons Why Mental Illness Still Has A Stigma

1. Not a lot of people are open to talking about it.

It can be very difficult to open up about an issue that is constantly made out to be a bad thing. Who would want to be open and honest about having a problem that will only result in being judged? The more that mental illness is brought up and discussed openly is the only way to spread further awareness and be made to see that it's not such a bad thing after all. The more it's brought up and understood, the more others may be willing to talk about it as well.

2. Mental illness is viewed as a weakness.

Many may think or view mental illness as a weakness. It's an illness, not a weakness or a personality flaw. The sooner people recognize this, the better. Those who live with a mental illness often possess many positive and artistic strengths such as higher IQ's, increased creativity (writing, art, music, etc), and greater empathy and compassion.

3. **Mental illness is portrayed negatively in the media.**

From the news, to articles, and in movies, mental illness has been labeled and seen as a "crazy disease" and whoever has one, must, in fact, be crazy and flawed. In the media, people with mental illnesses are often highlighted or portrayed as serial killers, violent, criminals, addicts/abusers, or just plain "crazy." In fact, did you know that those who live with a mental illness are more likely to be the victim in a crime or an abusive situation? In today's society, people are greatly influenced by what is in the media and mental illness isn't the only issue that is misunderstood or stereotyped. For example, many people, primarily women, think they should be skinny because it's *supposedly* viewed as more attractive or more acceptable. Another example would be homosexuality, in which some think being gay is a disease or a choice. Some fear it and show ignorance towards the homosexual community just like they do with mental illness, but think of how hurt a person could be to be judged or hated for something that isn't in their control. It's all in how the brain operates. There is no choice or fault.

4. **Some may be ashamed or are in denial of their own mental health.**

Some may feel embarrassed to have an illness, which is not a bad thing because this may be due to the stigma and how others view and react to mental illness. As a result, those with mental illness feel ashamed and may not feel comfortable talking about it. No one wants to viewed as the person who has a "problem" or to be thought of as less of a person for it especially when it's not true. The best thing to do for a person with mental illness is to listen and let them know that it is okay to talk about it.

5. People don't see mental illness as an important issue in our society.

There are not enough people to stand up for this particular issue in our society. Not enough people see this as an issue which is unfortunate because everyone will or has experienced some form of mental health issue. Anxiety, mood disorders, depression, eating disorders, and addictions, are some examples of mental health issues.

6. Some may be judgmental.

Those who may be appear judgmental just lack understanding and knowledge on the issue. Some judge out of fear because they don't understand it. Maybe informing or helping others understand is the answer.

How to overcome the stigma?

Read up more on mental illness, improve education on mental health, research, and try to change the outlook on mental health. Most of all, reach out, speak out, and promote awareness!

BONUS Material: Poetry and Writing By the Author

I Have An Illness. I Am Not Crazy...

I am a person who lives with bipolar disorder.

Does this scare you or perhaps make you think twice about the person I am?

Before you judge me based on my illness, there are some things I would like you to know.

I am not insane.

I am not acting out for attention.

I have a chemical imbalance in my brain that alters the emotions and how I feel.

I cannot control how I feel and act occasionally.

I am not violent.

I have never been involved in any crimes.

I have never hurt anyone physically.

People with bipolar disorder just want to be loved and accepted as everyone else does.

We want the same things for ourselves as others do.

We have goals.

We want to succeed.

We have many of the same interests and desires.

We are human.

How does a "label" such as bipolar disorder make us less than?

Try listening, understanding, and education first.

You may be surprised…

Bipolar is nothing like how it is portrayed in the media.

Never judge anything that is not clearly understood.

Don't judge at all.

I have an illness…

I am not crazy.

Things Are Never As They Appear to Be

Happy, delightful, sensitive child.

A girl with a wild imagination and endless dreams.

A girl with no worries?

Not at all.

How could she be expected to stand so tall?

With fearful images disturbing her mind.

She wasn't so happy all of the time.

Did she seem perfect from afar?

A girl with a bright future that has it all?
Happy turned sad, insecure, adolescent.
Anxiety, stress, and loneliness.
Insecurity and pain filled her veins.
Oh, the self-hatred, the anxiety remains.
Time and again, she felt alone.
She longed to be accepted, perhaps to be saved.
With no one by her side
-She wish she had died.
Maybe they would finally listen.
Maybe they would finally see.
All the pain I had kept within me.
Me?
Why, yes.
Who else would it be?
I'm far from perfect
-I'm a catastrophe.
Can't you see?
Things are never as they appear to be…

True Friends
Throughout life,
Friends may turn on you.

-Or you may turn on them.

You'll discover who is honest and true

-And those that never failed to fool you.

A true friend is someone you can trust.

-But who also forgives.

A person who brings out the best.

-And is supportive during the worst.

Never forget who your true friends are.

-No matter how close

-No matter how far.

I Used To Know A Guy.

I used to know a guy who envied, controlled, and deceived.

He raged whenever he was unhappy.

To gain control.

To frighten.

To seem bigger than me.

Inside I was dying.

I never knew why I stayed as long as I had.

There was a fear to let go and I never understood why.

I was afraid.

I felt alone.

I had isolated myself away from my family and people

who actually cared about me.

I lost contacts with friends.

I was crying on the inside and outside.

I hated who I was.

I lost all confidence in myself.

I made our relationship seem ideal when it really wasn't.

I stuck up for him when he never deserved it.

I wanted to be saved from this nightmare.

I admit though, not everyday was terrible like described.

He had a switch.

One direction was a more tolerable side of him.

The other direction was hell.

He found reasons or excuses to leave.

He would start fights, loud arguments, and yell at me.

Making me feel worthless..

I always got the blame.

He had to make himself look better.

"She did this"

"She started it"

"she made me feel this"

"she hit me"

"she's calling me names"

Often, very childish claims..

Sometimes, I had actually done some of those things to him.

I would scream, turn into a monster, just to feel or have some sense of control.

I wasn't myself, but I felt I had no other choice.

I had to protect myself.

I am not a monster, but he made me feel like one.

Did he ever tell the truth?

Did anyone ever know that he would yell at the top of his lungs in my face?

Block door ways so I couldn't exit?

Follow me around the house and refuse to give me space?

Threatening me ("If you do that I'll screw you over twice as bad")?

Threaten to leave and be able to come back as he pleases?

Talk badly about me?

Make up stories about me?

Using my family and I?

Overly jealous and belittling me?

After all that, he still expected me to take him back.

Over and over again.

He would apologize and then find ways to reel me

back in.

Most of the time he would never acknowledge that he had done anything wrong.

It was a constant battle.

A game.

A game that I no longer wanted to play.

He started a yelling match for the last time and said he was leaving once again.

I told him "This is the last time and I am not taking you back after this."

I meant it.

He called about a month or two later.

Sent e-mails.

He wanted to come back.

He said he was sorry and that he knows he treated me badly.

He wondered why I didn't want to talk to him.

I began talking to him for a while only to break the news that I was taken.

He couldn't believe that I had found a nice guy.

Why was that so hard to believe?

I refused to be just an option when I could be someone's whole world.

This new guy actually loves me for who I am.

There isn't anything he wouldn't do for me.

If I have a bad day, he helps me cope.

He keeps me strong.

He gave me my confidence back.

He treats me how a lady deserves to be treated.

He shows me what love really is.

I used to know a guy who never deserved me in the first place…

Now I am happy to be with a gentleman who most certainly does.

The Soul He Loves

I cannot bear to look him in the eyes, for he will know the truth of what I am.

My stomach in knots.

My heart is pounding.

My mind is racing, clouded with fear.

Little did I know, this love must be real…

The way he smiles leaves me guessing.

Forever wondering what he sees.

Is there something on my face?

What about me could he possibly embrace?

I'm far from perfect.

I'm blunt as can be.

I'm not like the other girls you may normally see.

I have an odd sense of humor.

I wear my heart on my sleeve.

I am as loyal as can be until you ask me to leave.

I over-think and over-analyze every little thing.

I'm a careless girl with a million dreams.

I am a mess of chaos spiraling out of control.

Yet he proceeds to love my soul.

Unstable – A Look into a Bipolar Mood Swing

A stable day turned quickly into an unstable night. Fear emerged within her, she suddenly felt alone. Feelings of emptiness, insanity, and confusion took over the girl I once knew. Within seconds, only her desperate cries out for help were left to be heard. She took her shaking hands as tears streamed endlessly upon her cheeks and placed them firmly over her head. She gripped her head tightly as she continued to rock back and forth. "I'm scared" she cried. I didn't know why. I didn't know what to do. I was lost and angered that I couldn't help her. "What do I do," I thought to myself. I began to think fast. To think of anything that may soothe her pain. I immediately reached over and held her tightly as I could. I didn't let go. She cried out a bit louder and started digging her nails into the bed that we were sitting upon. I was confused and unsure of what to do. The last thing I wanted to do was upset her even more. She wasn't able to verbalize what she needed or what was wrong at that point. She thought I didn't love her – My heart was breaking at that moment. "What did I do?" "I must have done something wrong." I thought to myself once again. The only thing I could do was be there for her, but I felt as if that wasn't enough. Her needs were unclear and I was beginning to quickly tire. She seemed to grow even more uncomfortable as I drifted to sleep. "Don't leave me." "Stay with me," she said. I couldn't understand. "I'm here. I'm not going anywhere. I love you," I said to her as I remained confused. Her cries began to soften as she looked back at me with her glossy eyes. "But you won't be here if you fall asleep," she said. With even more confusion, I looked at her for a couple of minutes, speechless. It became even more frustrating as she became increasingly angry and began crying out again. I couldn't understand why and I didn't know how to help her…

It was one trigger leading to the next. It was those unexpected moments that turned a pleasant, productive day into a nightmare. I never have understood myself and why I seem to act the way I do. I became increasingly shaken up and agitated. I began to cry out from the discomfort of the feelings within. Feeling scared and alone, I felt the uneasiness spiraling in the pit of my stomach. I began rocking back and forth as I held my head with the palms of my hands and fingertips. It was an unusual way that I would try to comfort myself. He looked at me with great confusion-he looked annoyed. I began to cry out from the fears within. I was fearing what he was thinking and feeling about me at this moment. I didn't have a clue. I remained irritable as I began making a complete fool of myself. I couldn't explain to him clearly enough why I was feeling this way or what was going on. He started to drift into sleep as I could see that he was exhausted. I became hostile as I repeatedly told him that I needed him with me at that moment. I felt incredibly selfish. I was afraid of being alone and I really needed him, but that didn't feel like a good enough excuse. I'm an adult and I should be able to take care of myself. My thoughts were swarming about in my mind as I became confused and unsure of what I wanted anymore. I shut him out as a quick defense- I didn't know what else to do. The last thing I would want is to hurt him because I love him and he deserves the best. Why should he have to put up with this? I began to dig my fingernails on the surface of the sheets as I became increasingly maddened by those thoughts. I remained frustrated and I could see that he was as well. He reached over to me and held me firmly in his arms. I could feel the tears streaming down my face onto his shoulder. As he held me I felt a sense of security. He's not going anywhere. He's here with me. I wasn't quickly soothed, but I was beginning to be reassured. I could tell his confusion grew with each minute passing. My only wish at that time was that he could understand the situation, for I could not explain what was happening. I didn't want him to hate or become angry with me. All these worries made the fears, crying out, and thoughts to continue. I wanted this moment to quickly pass. I want to be my best self and I don't want this to define me in any way. My hope is that he can understand…

The Author's Story

Ever since I were a young child I had been experiencing abnormal amounts of anxiety. I suffered with obsessive and intrusive thoughts as well as separation anxiety. It was terrifying to experience as a young child, but it was all I had ever known. I didn't know any better. At night, I would almost never sleep. I had an over-active imagination, racing thoughts, and fears of going to school. There were many times that I just did not attend school due to the extreme amounts of anxiety and discomfort. Around age 8, my parents took me to see a psychiatrist and therapist because they knew that something just wasn't right. The first psychiatrist and therapist I had seen weren't helpful and didn't see anything wrong with the behaviors I had been exhibiting. When my parents took me to see another psychiatrist for a second opinion, he determined a diagnosis after a couple of years of trying different medications to see the effectiveness. I was then diagnosed at age 12 with bipolar NOS (rapid-cycling) and a severe anxiety disorder.

It seemed like after the diagnosis is when the disorder worsened. My teen years were a living hell and it felt as though they were wasted with doctors appointments, consuming dozens of medications, hospitalizations , and feelings of emptiness and worthlessness. It seemed like those years of pain and struggling would last forever. It wasn't until after high school, which was a huge struggle for me, that I began to mellow out some and try to take control of my life.

Today, I haven't done this well in a very long while or ever. I am living independently with my boyfriend, my two cats, and a ferret. I feel as though I can finally start to live and enjoy my life which was very difficult for me to do previously. About a year ago, I started experiencing mixed episodes. That has been one of my main struggles at this point in time. There will be some really crummy days where I won't feel like or just can't do much at all. I try to rest and wait out the low moments and try to keep in mind that they don't last forever. The mania isn't too severe, but at times I do get very hyper, I talk a mile a minute, I laugh constantly, sometimes I want to spend money, and I have a quite a bit of anxiety and worries. Things haven't been terribly unmanageable lately though and I am very thankful for that.

www.ingramcontent.com/pod-product-compliance
Lightning Source LLC
Chambersburg PA
CBHW051255170526
45165CB00004B/1727